Weight Loss Exercises

Awesome Fat Burn

Table of Contents

Weight Loss Exercises 1

Awesome Fat Burn 1

Get Rid Of Those Pesky Extra Pounds 5

Cardio Exercises - Universal Solution for Health, Heart, Diabetes and Obesity..8

Ways To Burn More Fat 11

Novice Cardio Training 15

How to Lose Weight Fast 19

A How-To Guide For Six Pack Abs 21

Cardio for Weight Loss - 3 Best Cardio Exercises That Helps You Lose Weight 24

These are some of my other books below, and my website is
www.LosingBellyFatMission.com :

https://www.amazon.com/dp/B06XB4WHZX
http://www.amazon.com/dp/B06X9LXBB8
http://www.amazon.com/dp/B06WLK7497
http://www.amazon.com/dp/B06W54JKQN
http://www.amazon.com/dp/B06X6DJ9K3
http://www.amazon.com/dp/B06WGNJ9N3
http://www.amazon.com/dp/B06W549TBD
http://www.amazon.com/dp/B06VTF5DQJ
http://www.amazon.com/dp/B06WRPSBKK
http://www.amazon.com/dp/B06WD194JR
http://www.amazon.com/dp/B06WCZTK7Y
http://www.amazon.com/dp/B06X3QN1HT
http://www.amazon.com/dp/B01N19WBF2
http://www.amazon.com/dp/B01N2AVECA
http://www.amazon.com/dp/B01N4VZIAV
http://www.amazon.com/dp/B00QJJFS1C
http://www.amazon.com/dp/B01EMNO2MW
http://www.amazon.com/dp/B00SSFWCPA
http://www.amazon.com/dp/1520531230
http://www.amazon.com/dp/B01N4V7SR9
http://www.amazon.com/dp/B00SX58DUI
http://www.amazon.com/dp/B010K7YP62
http://www.amazon.com/dp/B012LAYNNQ

http://www.amazon.com/dp/B00RVX3KY2
http://www.amazon.com/dp/B01MR6SWGW
http://www.amazon.com/dp/B00XF6G4HO
http://www.amazon.com/dp/B01F1472N2
http://www.amazon.com/dp/B00PQ0TUPU
http://www.amazon.com/dp/B00PP8OZJ4
http://www.amazon.com/dp/B00QH7DY4Y
http://www.amazon.com/dp/B01052010G
http://www.amazon.com/dp/B00QDHXN7Q
http://www.amazon.com/dp/B00PO0IQIO

Among others.

Get Rid Of Those Pesky Extra Pounds

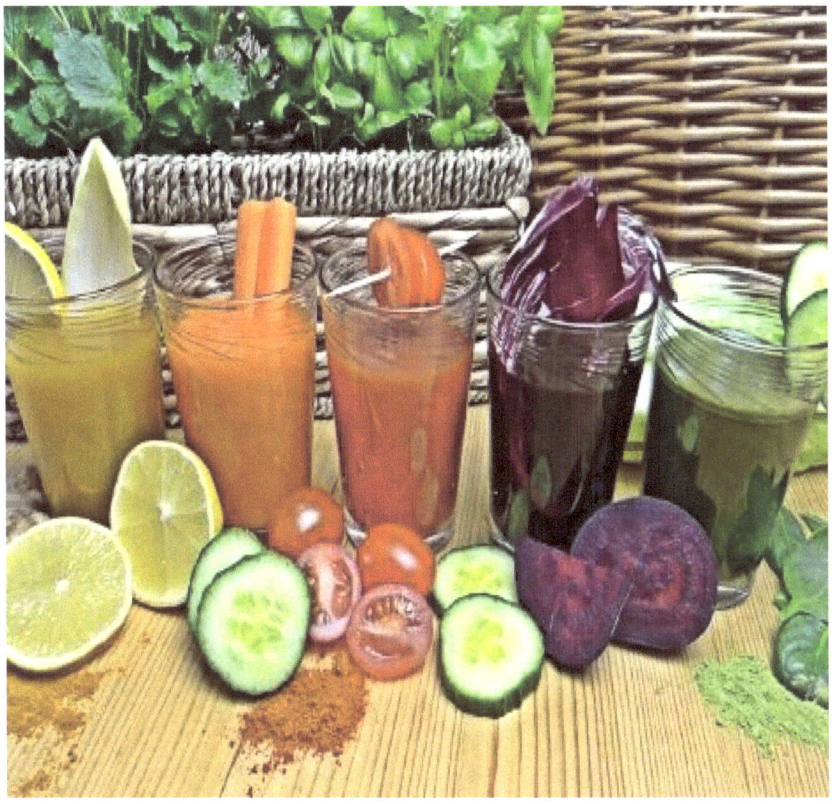

Losing weight isn't always easy especially for those suffering from obesity. But that definitely doesn't mean that you should give up. Most people adopt various methods in order to lose their weight rapidly and in their pursuit of losing it fast, they end up gaining more and more. Some are so much desperate that they start utilizing silly techniques or tips, but they are merely a waste of time for them and in the end they just loose hope. Instead of relying on the idea and belief that they can lose a significant amount of weight in a month or fifteen days, they should follow some basic and effective strategies or tips to lose it in a healthy manner that takes time but is always fruitful in the long run. There are countless techniques and methods that a person can adopt for losing weight or shedding some extra pounds the faster and healthier way.

Some of these efficient techniques are detailed below: One of the most effective ways to lose weight fast is to perform intense cardio exercises daily. Although these strong cardio exercises are advantageous for the body and its better functioning yet too much exercise without an interval for relaxation can be detrimental for the body too. So, by adding a little twist to the normal cardio routine, you can bring amazingly huge changes towards accomplishing your objective of losing weight rapidly. This change in your regular hourly exercise is a ten to fifteen minute break. This break time is quite crucial because it helps elevate your metabolic rate faster and for a longer duration as compared to a tiring and continuous cardio workout. Taking a small break for rest is always healthy for your body and mind and can help you lose incremental weight in the long run. Applying this strategy in your daily intense workout routine can be quite beneficial for you in the future.

One of the most effective cardio exercises include walking, running or cycling. Participating in any of these activities will cause huge positive changes towards your health and will definitely help your body lose weight quickly. Applying stress on the liver for performing the function of the kidneys is not a good idea at all. Therefore, it's best that you drink lots and lots of water daily for the better functioning of your kidneys. If your kidneys are unable to perform efficiently due to slackness in drinking water then this can be a huge problem for your health in the long run. Drinking at least six or eight glasses of water daily is essential for your health and it also aids towards elevating the metabolic rate of your body. By increasing the metabolic rate of your body, you enable your body to break up and use the stored fats of the body. This helps a lot in shedding extra pounds. Apart from the regular and timely intake of fresh water, your nutrition also plays a deciding role towards weight gain. The more you incline towards fast foods and unhealthy nutrition, the more is the likelihood of you damaging your health and gaining unnecessary weight. So, it's best that you avoid greasy and artificially sweetened foods and tend towards healthy foods which include fresh salads, vegetables and above all fresh and juicy fruits. These healthy food items help a lot towards making your digestive system function in a much better way. On the other hand, fast food items which include burgers, fried chips or pizza items lead toward the intake of dangerous amount of calories and in the end you only drag yourself in a direction that makes your liver fatty and lazy towards performing its basic function. Moreover you should try to develop the habit of drinking more and more green tea and eat more and more fibers and proteins. Moreover, skipping breakfast isn't a good idea at all and will only cause health problems. Your body automatically burns more calories in the morning than other times of the day. Therefore, you should eat a healthy breakfast without worries.

Cardio Exercises - Universal Solution for Health, Heart, Diabetes and Obesity

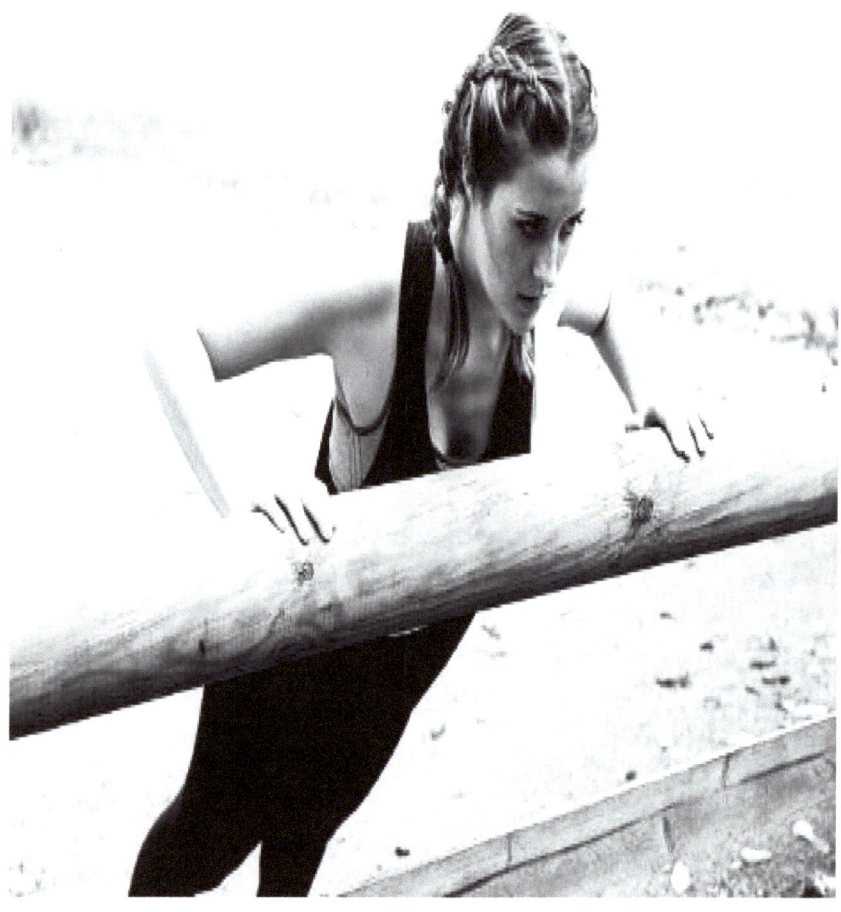

If you want to provide continuous exercise for all your muscle groups in the body at the same time, there is none better than Cardio exercises.

Making a success of cardio training depends on how effectively it can elevate your heart rate (an increase of 60 to 80% would be a good figure) and improve the muscles in your heart. The major physical exercises that form part of cardiovascular training will include jogging, running, walking, swimming, cycling, rowing and even aerobic exercises. Consistent pursuit of cardio training can promote a healthy body and mind in the end. Please see below some of the benefits accruing from cardio training. Energy levels A boost in your energy levels is the first benefit from regularly performing cardio exercises like jogging, swimming, running, or aerobics.

Constant and habitual cardio training will adapt your body to endure more exercise regimes as time goes by, and you will feel more energized and less tired when doing more strenuous work. Cardio workouts are ideal to increase your physical endurance levels. Metabolism Consistency and regularity in cardio workouts offer enhanced body metabolism. Since the cardio workouts strengthen the heart muscles, they are able to cope with the extra strain resulting in the body burning more calories in an efficient manner. The increased metabolism of the body helps to manage the additional energy required due to increased physical activity. Regular cardiovascular exercises help the body to maintain their increased metabolism rate, consequently burning extra calories and conveniently resulting in loss of weight. Weight control Regular Cardio training is a great boon to avid weight loss aspirants, who dream to keep their weight constant at a particular level. The higher metabolism that results from cardio training burns up calories faster and helps in burning up the stored body fats. The universal physical activity rendered by cardio training helps to build up the body muscles.

Loss of weight is a positive benefit from cardio workouts, which, if done continuously, will also help you to maintain your weight in the long haul. How it helps the heart as mentioned above, regular cardio exercises strengthen the heart muscles, thereby increasing the heart's efficiency. With the new-found muscle strength, the heart grows stronger and becomes immune to the diseases that threaten it. Cardio exercises, in addition to providing a healthy heart, also make your lungs stronger. Performing cardio workouts regularly have benefits for diseases like obesity, diabetes and even those concerning the heart. In the final analysis, we can conclude that cardio exercises favorably contribute to reduced levels of stress and risk of diseases, provides relief from anxiety, helps you to sleep better, energizes your body and most importantly encourage your kids into following in your cardio footsteps.

Ways To Burn More Fat

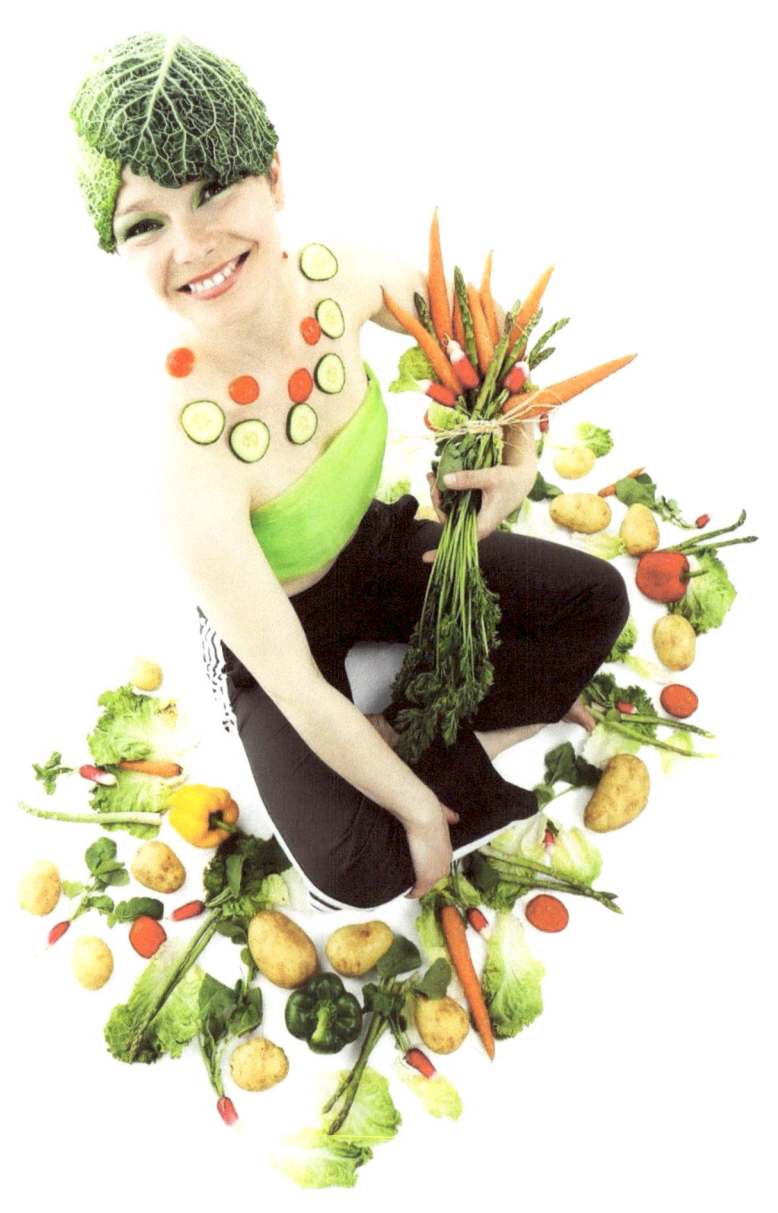

There are many ways to lose weight. So here are some ways in which you can burn more body fat to achieve the figure that you desire. Increase Muscle Mass - One of the best way to burn more fat is to increase your body's muscle mass by training with weights. This is because the more muscle you have, the more calories your body will burn even when you are sleeping. This is because muscle is extremely active metabolically and the foods that you eat will need to feed your muscle instead of being stored as body fat. Girls are often afraid to gain muscle because they think that they will look like The Incredible Hulk. Ladies, rest be assured that you will not look like professional female bodybuilders for a number of reasons. On the contrary, the muscles that you gain will give you the healthy well toned sexy look once you have gotten rid of your excess body fat.

Avoid Poor Quality Carbs - Eat less poor quality carbohydrates commonly known as high glycemic carbs, especially before bed. These are carbs that are easily digestible like sugar, white bread, cereals, mashed potatoes, pastas etc. These carbs spike up your insulin level in your bloodstream pretty quickly and cause your body to store body fat.

Never Skip Meals - Do you skip meals, especially breakfast? Don't do that. That is not the right way of consuming fewer calories. When you skip meals and go hungry, your body will simply react in a way that there is a scarcity of food and it will protect you by storing your body fat and burning your muscle for energy. Your metabolism will plummet into the abyss. Furthermore, when you are starving, you will probably be eating more at your next meal and in turn eating more calories than required and thus putting on even more fat.

Cardio Variations - If you are doing cardio exercises to burn calories and fat, it may be a good idea that from time to time split your cardio training into two short sessions rather than one long one. Numerous studies have shown that people who do 30 minutes of cardio in the morning and then 30 minutes in the evening lose more fat than those doing just one hour duration cardio exercises at a stretch. There is a science to this, but that is for another article.

Alcohol Abstinence - Avoid alcohol. Alcohol is not only harmful to your body, it also chock full of calories at 7 calories per gram. Furthermore, people usually drink alcohol with a cocktail of sugary drinks adding even more calories.

Beauty Sleep - Do you have enough sleep? Sleep deprivation will upset your hormonal balance and suppresses fat burning hormones such as testosterone and human growth hormone or HGH. A lack of sleep also put your body into stress and thus increases the production of cortisol, a hormone that is known to store body fat.

Consume Fiber - Do eat plenty of high fiber foods such as vegetables, especially crucible vegetables like broccoli and cauliflower. Fibers not only promote overall general health, but also significantly aid in the fat-burning process. By just following the fat burning ways suggested in this article, you will be burning more fat than you know and soon, you will see positive results right before your very eyes.

Novice Cardio Training

BODYWEIGHT WORKOUT

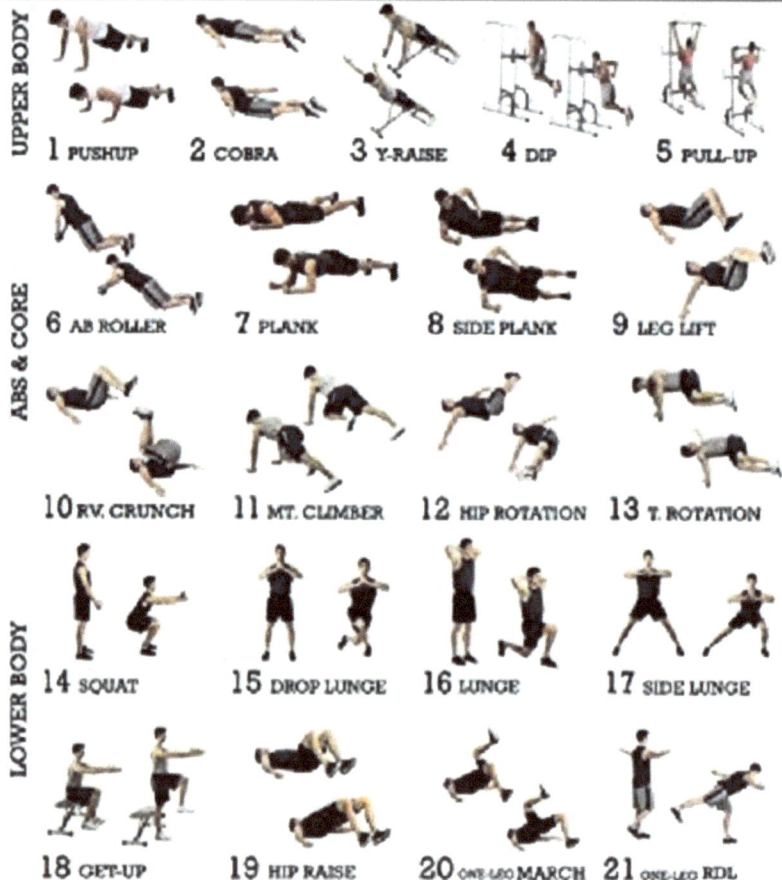

UPPER BODY

1 PUSHUP 2 COBRA 3 Y-RAISE 4 DIP 5 PULL-UP

ABS & CORE

6 AB ROLLER 7 PLANK 8 SIDE PLANK 9 LEG LIFT

10 RV. CRUNCH 11 MT. CLIMBER 12 HIP ROTATION 13 T. ROTATION

LOWER BODY

14 SQUAT 15 DROP LUNGE 16 LUNGE 17 SIDE LUNGE

18 GET-UP 19 HIP RAISE 20 ONE-LEG MARCH 21 ONE-LEG RDL

REPS	10-15	2-4
SETS	REPETITIONS	SETS

Are you a cardio training novice? Don't feel insecure, because there are many people just like you! Developing a cardio routine that is actually effective isn't an easy task. Yes, you can go and run miles after miles, but let's be honest, that doesn't work. Old school aerobic training that is not only boring, but ineffective will not provide you with the long term gains you're looking for. This is why you must focus your energy on high-intensity cardio. Don't be afraid. Once you start, you will never go back to boring cardio exercises again! High-intensity cardio exercises are challenging, but the rewards are huge. Instead of spending 60 minutes on a treadmill, you will now only need to spend 20-30 minutes at the gym. Within this 20 or 30-minute timeframe, you are guaranteed to burn twice as many calories as you would with a long aerobic routine.

So what exercises should you use? Bodyweight Exercises Meatheads used to advise against bodyweight exercises because of the exercises' "ineffective". Like I said, they are meatheads. Bodyweight exercises are an excellent cardio option for incinerate fat, and building lean muscle at the same time. The best part, is that there are hundreds of different exercises you can utilize to develop an effective regime. The most popular workouts include squat variations, push-up variations, burpees, mountain climbers, planks, and plank walks. Anyone can develop their very own routine by finding, and putting together a group of exercises. It's really simple, but very effective.

Sprints

A personal favorite of mine. Sprints are one the best fat burning cardio exercises you can use. When it comes to high-intensity, sprints take the crown. A typical sprint regime will take about 15-20 minutes to complete, and you will burn a massive amount of calories. I recommend not sprinting any longer than 60-yards because it will not only disrupt your running form, but you are likely to slow down and not be able to maintain 100 percent intensity for distance longer. Also, distances longer than 60 yards may force your body in an aerobic state, which is not the purpose of sprints. Traditional sprints are incredibly effective, but to up the ante, you can try hill sprints, interval sprints, or resistance sprints. Each exercise increases the difficulty, but should only be used once you have mastered the traditional version. These are only a few of the many cardio exercises you can use to achieve great fat loss results, but you can also include plyometrics, agility's, and interval training into the mix. High-intensity cardio exercises will always triumph over low-intensity!

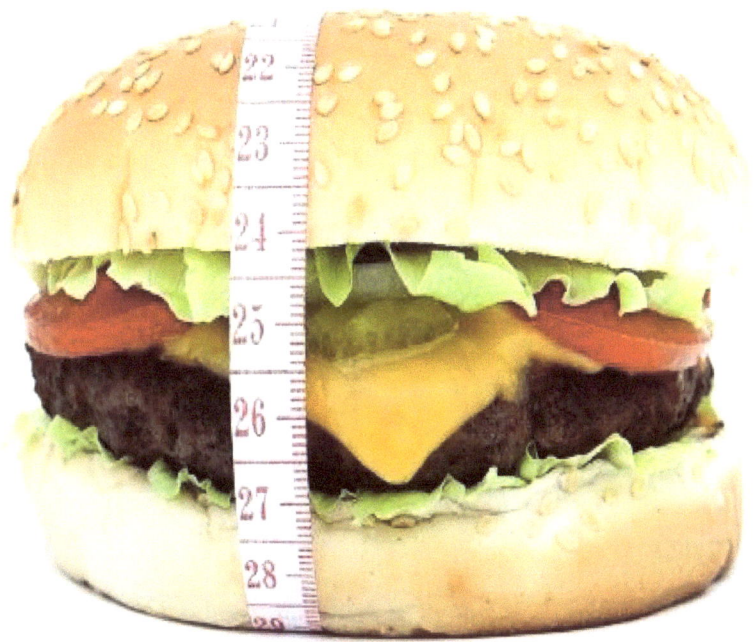

First it is wise to think if this is good to lose weight in a fast way. In many cases it could be dangerous for your health and typically you will gain fat again. It doesn't mean that it is not possible. Don't starve yourselves but eat less than before and eat more often. Don't eat fat meals, only boiled meat and vegetables. The most important thing is to drink a lot of water. Thanks to water you will not be so hungry. Drink at least 8 glasses of water. Eat slowly, don't speed up and carefully chew your meal. Have fun from every piece of your meal. Eat lot of food that consist water like tomatoes, water melons, grapes etc. Try fat burning soups. They are very good because they contain a lot of water food and also fat burning food. Eat breakfast. They are the most important meal during the day. Don't eat after 8 pm. Be careful about fat and carbohydrates that are in your meal. Try to decrease them. Eat more protein which burns fat while being burned.

Make exercises for example stomach crunches or other. Do them a lot including cardio exercises like running, biking, swimming or tennis. Cardio exercises are very god for lowering fat from your body. If you have a dog, walk with him longer then usually if not do walking as well. Buy yourself a pedometer and count your walk. You should make 10 000 steps a day and it is not that difficult. Try to walk or use a bike to get to your work place instead of using a car. With exercises you have to be systematic and if you do them for 3 weeks you will see the difference. Go to a gym. People tend to participate in things that they paid for. You can support your diet with some diet pills. Consult it with your doctor.

Don't drink alcohol. Believe it or not but alcohol has a lot of calories. Sleep regularly and more then usually. Exercises can be very exhausted so give yourself a chance to recover after training but not too long. When you are rested you have more strength to continue with your fight against the fat. Reword yourself after each 2-3 weeks of hard training and diet by buying some nice things for yourself. This will motivate you. Buy a trip to sunny place with beaches were you can be proud of your new look. Loosing weight fast can be hard and dangerous but it is possible and can be safe for people that want to loss weight fast.

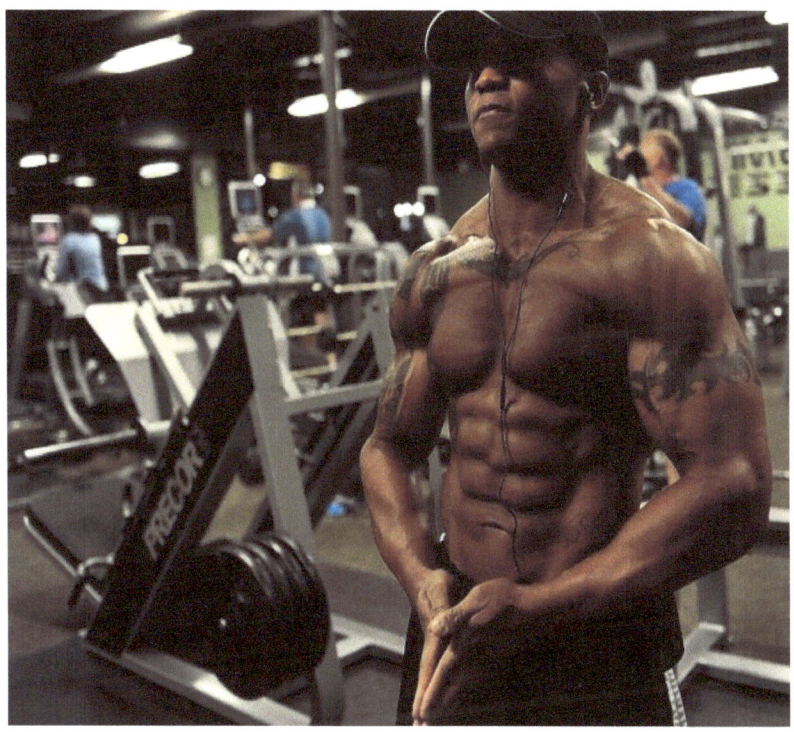

Getting six pack abs is no mean feat, but in order to really get your abs as protruding and defined as possible, it's important that you are able to do the methods and techniques which work quickly and effectively. We've found that there are a lot of poor quality tutorials out there, and we want to set the record straight with this one:

Step 1 - Nutrition & Diet The first step to getting six pack abs is to get your diet under control. Many people have stomach fat covering their abs, making it essential that you limit the amount of fat on your body. And to do this, you need to make sure that your body has a "high metabolism" rate. Metabolism is the mechanism inside your body which controls how much fat is kept on your arms, legs, stomach and neck. The "higher" your metabolism, the less fat your body will store, allowing you to burn it off easier and quicker. It's important to get a high metabolism so that you can burn off your body fat and reveal the abs underneath. And do this, there are certain "rules" you need to follow: Never eat the same amount (calories) of food each day. Vary it according to "Calorie Cycling" techniques. This will boost your metabolism Eat only wholesome, nutritious food (no microwave meals or McDonald's) Stick to eating 3 set meals a day resist the temptation to snack on junk Drink plenty of water (so you need to pee at least 3 times a day) Make sure you eat breakfast as this will set your metabolism up well for the rest of the day. You will also want to eat these kinds of foods: Whole Grains Fruits Vegetables Chicken Fish Lots of protein Eggs Nuts Water Milk (has calcium).

Step 2 - Exercise Once you have your diet under control, it's time to perform the exercises which are going to burn off your stomach fat and make your abs protrude. There are a lot of exercises out there, but let me make it crystal clear that doing sit ups will not burn fat from your stomach. The exercise routines you need to follow should fall into a pattern. There are cardiovascular exercises (such as running, walking, swimming and cycling) which will burn fat. These exercises are essential as a "foundation" for your abs. The other set of exercises you need to do focus purely on building the abdominal muscles, including such exercises as sit ups, crunches and push ups. Here are the typical exercises you should incorporate into your weekly routines: Fat Burning Exercises Multi-Jointed cardio exercises (great for fat burning) Running

Walking Swimming Aerobics classes Cycling Rowing Anything that gets you "hot & sweaty" Ab Toning Exercises Sit ups Crunches Inclined Sit Ups Russian Twists Leg Thrusts Lateral Pull-Downs Kettle Bell Exercises These exercises should be performed on different days in different amounts. The number one 'secret' to getting more powerful and bigger abs, is that challenging your body is VITAL.

The more you are able to challenge your body each day, the more it will have to change and adapt to meet your requirements; and that's where more muscle definition comes in and fat burning takes place. However, in order to see the most effective and fastest results, you need to be able to put all of these tips into a routine that works well to burn the most fat on your body and makes your abs more defined and protruding. I have been able to discover what works and what doesn't in my own quest to grow my own six-pack and have put all the best secrets on my site.

Cardio for Weight Loss - 3 Best Cardio Exercises That Helps You Lose Weight

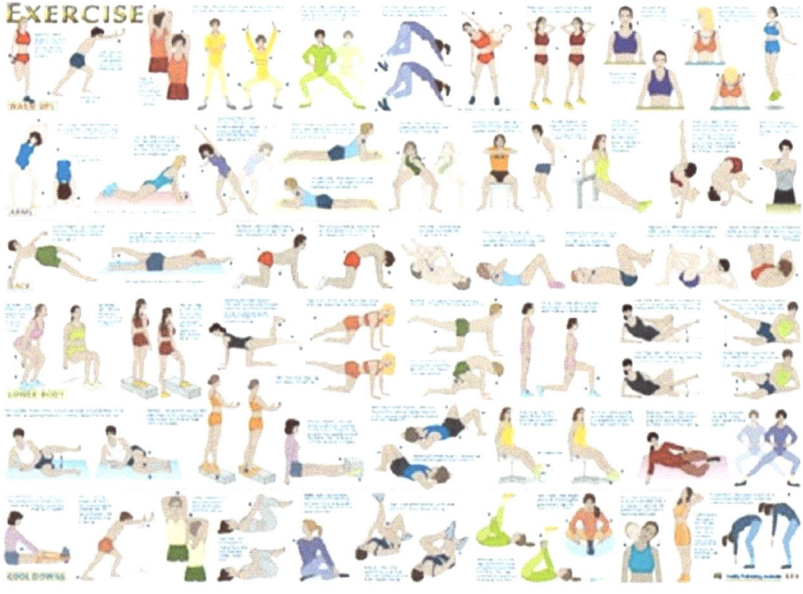

Cardio for weight loss is a very popular way for you to burn the pounds. This is because they make use of your arms and legs keeping you toned all over. It's also good for the heart so it keeps you away from health risks. But nowadays people don't believe in cardio for weight loss anymore claiming that they don't work. They say they're doing cardio for weight loss for months but they just didn't lose anything. This is because they only exercise for about 20 minutes every other day. What they don't know is that the fat burning process starts when you're doing 20 minutes of exercises so when you quit, the fat burning process stops too. They also do not increase their level of exercise keeping their exercise intensity to an average level. What's more is that they only exercise for two to three weeks.

It is recommended that you do a minimum of 45 minutes of cardio for weight loss exercises for 3-4 times a week to get real weight loss results. And you also have to challenge yourself, not just stay on the same speed all the time. That doesn't mean you'll be pushing yourself to the limit. And now that you know how long you'll be doing your cardio for weight loss and what are the tricks to be able to burn pounds with it, here are the 3 best cardio for weight loss exercises that have proven to make you lose weight:

1. Jogging

Everybody prefers jogging because it's the easiest thing to do. And that's about right. It also helps you lose fat in all the places as well. Not only does jogging makes you lose weight but it also tones your body giving you a lean and fit look. Jogging doesn't need to be in the gym with a treadmill. You can just jog in your neighborhood or at the park. Although you have to look out for your ankles and knees the most since you'll be using them a lot.

2. Bicycling

Bicycling is another type of cardio for weight loss exercise that is effective when it comes to losing weight. It also improves your sense of balance when you're riding at an average speed for an hour. The more leg power you put when you are riding will make you burn more calories. Bicycling will also strengthen your heart and just like jogging, it will also tone your body.

3. Swimming

If you don't like bicycling or jogging or you're just not the outdoors type then you might want to try swimming. Swimming uses both your arms and legs so you'll be able to lose the flabs in those areas that you've always wanted to get rid of. Swimming also strengthens the lungs and heart so you'll feel a healthier you when you're losing weight. Just like biking, the more you add speed to your strokes and kicks, the more you will be able to shed off pounds. These simple cardio for weight loss exercises are helpful when you want to slim down and when you have tried out one of these, you will find yourself agreeing to the same thing.

These are some of my other books below, and my website is
www.LosingBellyFatMission.com :

https://www.amazon.com/dp/B06XB4WHZX
http://www.amazon.com/dp/B06X9LXBB8
http://www.amazon.com/dp/B06WLK7497
http://www.amazon.com/dp/B06W54JKQN
http://www.amazon.com/dp/B06X6DJ9K3
http://www.amazon.com/dp/B06WGNJ9N3
http://www.amazon.com/dp/B06W549TBD
http://www.amazon.com/dp/B06VTF5DQJ
http://www.amazon.com/dp/B06WRPSBKK
http://www.amazon.com/dp/B06WD194JR
http://www.amazon.com/dp/B06WCZTK7Y
http://www.amazon.com/dp/B06X3QN1HT
http://www.amazon.com/dp/B01N19WBF2
http://www.amazon.com/dp/B01N2AVECA
http://www.amazon.com/dp/B01N4VZIAV
http://www.amazon.com/dp/B00QJJFS1C
http://www.amazon.com/dp/B01EMNO2MW
http://www.amazon.com/dp/B00SSFWCPA
http://www.amazon.com/dp/1520531230
http://www.amazon.com/dp/B01N4V7SR9
http://www.amazon.com/dp/B00SX58DUI
http://www.amazon.com/dp/B010K7YP62
http://www.amazon.com/dp/B012LAYNNQ
http://www.amazon.com/dp/B00RVX3KY2
http://www.amazon.com/dp/B01MR6SWGW

http://www.amazon.com/dp/B00XF6G4HO
http://www.amazon.com/dp/B01F1472N2
http://www.amazon.com/dp/B00PQ0TUPU
http://www.amazon.com/dp/B00PP8OZJ4
http://www.amazon.com/dp/B00QH7DY4Y
http://www.amazon.com/dp/B01052010G
http://www.amazon.com/dp/B00QDHXN7Q
http://www.amazon.com/dp/B00PO0IQIO

Among others.